ABC's of Nature's Best Herbal Recipes

Ombassa Sophera

ISBN-13: 978-1497300842

ISBN-10: 1497300843

DEDICATION

This book is dedicated to my Mom and Dad whose natural propensity for spiritual healing and emotional nurturing has gifted me with a legacy to love beyond all measure....I LOVE YOU BOTH!

ACKNOWLEDGMENTS

Special thanks to all of my children, Devonna, Darin, Devin and Devita and their children: Nia, DJ, Nailah, Dalil and Dakari for your love and support as I completed the process of delivering this book, my gift to the world.
Thanks Ade, for your committed support as my life friend and comrade.
I LOVE YOU ALL

ACCEPTANCE
Support for Diarrhea

1 cup Agrimony Leaf
1 cup Bilberry Leaf
2 tbl Cayenne Pepper
¼ cup Fenugreek Seed
1 cup Peppermint Leaf
1 cup Marshmallow Leaf
½ cup Pau D Arco Leaf
1 cup Raspberry Leaf
½ cup Strawberry Leaf
2 tbl Nutmeg

"I accept my life as it is right now"

ALL CLEAR
Support for Scars

2 Quarts Aloe Juice (non-acidic)
½ cup Comfrey Root
½ cup Black Walnut Leaf
1 cup Chamomile Flowers
1 cup Calendula Flowers
¼ cup Lavender Flowers

"I forgive and let it go."

APHRODISIAC
Support for the Sexual Organs

1 cup Ginseng Root
½ cup Cardamom Seed
3 tsp Nutmeg
½ cup Muira Puama
½ cup Horny Goat Weed
1 cup Fo-ti Root
1 cup Damania Leaf
½ cup Maca Root
½ cup Yohimbe Bark
½ cup Tribulus Terretris
¼ cup Tongkat Ali
1 cup Passionflower

"I am full of amazing, satisfying and powerful sexual energy"

ASSIMILATION
Support for Digestive Tract

½ cup Anise Seed
1 cup Parsley Leaf
1 cup Peppermint Leaf
½ cup Caraway Seed
½ cup Cardamom Seed
½ cup Fennel Seed
1 cup Marshmallow Leaf
1 cup Slippery Elm Bark
1 cup Chamomile Flowers
1 cup Lemon Balm Leaf
½ cup Gentian Root
½ cup Oregon Grape Root
½ cup Skullcap Leaf
½ cup Goldenseal Root
1 cup Wormwood Leaf

"With ease I assimilate what life has for me."

BETTER BREATH
Support for Bad Breath

½ cup Clove Bud
½ cup Anise Seed
½ cup Caraway Seed
½ cup Cardamom Seed
1 cup Parsley Leaf
1 cup Peppermint Leaf
½ cup Spearmint Leaf
¼ cup Wintergreen Leaf

"I allow a new attitude of sweetness to all"

BITTER SWEET
Support for the Stomach

1 cup Buchu Leaf
½ cup Fennel Seed
½ cup Ginger Root
1 cup Marshmallow Leaf
1 cup Slippery Elm Bark
1 cup Anise Seed
¼ cup Caraway Seed

"I effortlessly digest my life."

BLESS THE STRESS
Support for Adrenals

½ Licorice Root
1 cup Sarsaparilla Root
1 cup Bladderwrack Leaf
½ cup Irish Moss
½ cup Ginger Root
1 cup Astragalus Leaf
2 tbl Cayenne Pepper
1 cup Rose Hips Extract

"I take special care of me."

BOOST
Support for Immune System

½ cup Astragalus Root
½ cup Usnea Lichen
½ cup Sage Leaf
2 Juiced Bulbs of Garlic
½ cup Shitake Mushroom
½ cup Reishi Mushroom
1 cup Hyssop Leaf
1 cup St John's Wort Leaf
1 cup Bayberry Leaf
¼ cup Fenugreek Seeds
Quart Black Radish Juice
½ cup Dandelion Leaf
¼ cup Milk Thistle Seed
½ cup Boxthorn Dried Fruit
½ cup Ginseng Root
½ cup Wisteria Leaf
1 cup Echinacea Root
1 cup Echinacea Leaf
½ cup Licorice Root

"I am safe to now express and energized myself with joy!"

CHERISH ME
Support for Bruises

1 cup Bilberry Leaf
1 cup Stinging Nettle Leaf
1 cup Oat Straw
½ cup Ginger Root
1 cup Comfrey Root
½ cup Comfrey Leaf
¼ cup Lavender Flowers
½ cup Marjoram Leaf
1 cup Calendula Flowers

"Love is all I want, need and have. I'm now free to cherish me."

CHEW ON THAT
Support for the Mouth and Gums

¼ cup Myrrh Gum
2 Quarts Aloe Juice (non-acidic)
½ cup Clove Bud
1 cup Neem Leaf
1 cup Calendula Flowers
1 cup Peppermint Leaf
¼ cup Spearmint Leaf
1 cup Sage Leaf
1 cup Echinacea Root
1 cup White Oak Bark

"I choose. I support my decisions."

CHILLAX
Support for Anxiety

1 cup Kava Kava Root
½ cup Ginseng Leaf
½ cup Valerian Root
½ cup Lemon Balm Leaf
1 cup Catnip Leaf
¼ cup St John's Wort Leaf
1 cup Chamomile Flowers
¼ cup Lavender Flowers
½ cup Alfalfa Leaf
1 cup Peppermint Leaf
1 cup Oat Straw

"I no longer give my peace away to_____."

CLEAR AWAY
Support for Boils

Juice bulb of Garlic
Juice 12 Lemons
1 cup Goldenseal Leaf
½ cup Bladderwrack Leaf
1 cup Buchu Leaf
1 cup Echinacea Leaf
½ cup Echinacea Root
1 cup Alfalfa Leaf
¼ cup Rosemary Leaf
¼ cup Sage Leaf

"I am love, joy and peace."

CLEAR EAR
Support for Ear Infection

1 cup Echinacea Leaf

1 cup Elder Flowers

1 Whole Bulb Garlic

1 cup Alfalfa Leaf

1 cup Mullein Flowers

1 cup Goldenseal Leaf

½ cup Goldenseal Root

1 cup Olive Leaf

"I clear my ear to hear with love"

COOL RUNNINGS
Support as Anti-Inflammatory

1 cup Basil Leaf
1 cup Bergamot Leaf
½ cup Chamomile Flowers
1 cup Red Clover Leaf
1 cup Echinacea Leaf
½ cup Ginger Root
½ cup Rosemary Leaf
1 cup Yarrow Leaf
1 cup Sorrel Blossoms
½ cup Sheep Sorrel Leaf

"I release the hurt, anger and transmute it into love."

COURAGE
Support for Nausea

1 cup Anise Seed
¼ Fennel Seed
2 tbl Oregano Leaf
2 tbl Thyme
1 Bay Leaf
1 tsp Cayenne Pepper
1 cup Ginger Root
2 cups Peppermint Leaf
½ cup Goldenseal Leaf
3 tbl Nutmeg

"I have the courage to love beyond my fears."

CREATIVITY
Support for Tonsillitis

1 cup White Oak Bark
1 cup Witch Hazel Leaf
½ cup White Willow Bark
1 cup Goldenseal Leaf
1 cup Echinacea Leaf

"I freely express my creativity."

DEFENSE
Support as an Anti-Oxidant

20 Lemons
½ cup Turmeric Root
Pinch of Cayenne Pepper
1 cup Echinacea Root
1 cup Echinacea Leaf
½ cup Goldenseal Root
1 cup Goldenseal Leaf
1 cup Elder Berries
1 cup Sorrel Blossoms

"My love is a POWERFUL defense for anything I may encounter in life."

DIVINE MIND
Support for the Brain

1 cup Gotu Kola Leaf
1 cup Asian Ginseng Root
1 cup Siberian Ginseng Root
1 cup Guarana Berry
1 cup Gingko Leaf
½ cup Rosemary Leaf
1 cup Raspberry Leaf
1 cup Peppermint Leaf
½ cup Pennywort Leaf
½ cup Club Moss

"I enhance my cells and use every part of my brain."

DRY PANTS
Support for Bedwetting

Honey to taste
½ cup Oak Bark
1 cup Catmint Leaf
½ cup Uva Ursi Leaf
½ cup Horsetail Leaf
1 cup Mullein Flowers
½ cup Plantain Leaf
1 quart Cranberry Juice
1 cup Corn Silk

"I am supported and secure in love."

EASY NOW
Support for Congestion

½ cup Horseradish Root
½ cup Ginger Root
20 Squeezed Lemons
1 cup Comfrey Root
1 cup Elecampane Root
1 cup Slippery Elm Bark
½ cup Eucalyptus Leaf
1 cup Horehound Leaf
1 cup Hyssop Leaf
½ cup Pleurisy Root
¼ cup Thyme Leaf
½ cup Alfalfa Leaf
1 cup Mullein Flowers
1 cup Coltsfoot Leaf
½ cup Violet Leaf
¼ cup Cayenne Pepper
1 cup Peppermint Leaf
¼ cup Spearmint Leaf

"I allow my emotions to flow free into complete release."

EMANCIPATION
Support for Irritable Bowel Syndrome

½ cup Milk Thistle Seed
Quart of Aloe Juice (non-acidic)
1 cup Alfalfa Leaf
1 cup Marshmallow Leaf
1 cup Slippery Elm Bark
1 cup Peppermint Leaf
¼ cup Asafetida Powder
1 cup Chamomile Flowers
½ cup Cramp Bark
½ cup Cascara Sagrada Bark

"I release old, decrepit ideas."

ENCOURAGEMENT
Support with Varicose Veins

½ cup Horse Chestnut Leaf
½ cup Gotu Kola Leaf
1 cup Butchers Broom leaf
1 cup Witch Hazel Leaf
1 cup Violet Leaf
1 cup Calendula Flowers

"I live my truth and circulate my joy freely."

ENERGY
Support to Boost Energy

½ cup Ashwagandha
1 cup Yerba Mate Leaf
¼ cup Korean Ginseng Root
½ Eleuthero Root (Siberian Ginseng)
¼ cup Ginger Root
½ cup Green Tea
½ cup Ginkgo Root
1 cup Alfalfa Leaf

"I claim my massive measure of God-given energy."

EXCEPTIONAL BALANCE
Support for Kidneys

1 cup Artichoke Leaf
¼ cup Birch Bark
½ cup Borage Leaf
1 cup Buchu Leaf
½ cup Dandelion Root
½ cup Eleuthero Root
½ cup Fo-ti Root
1 cup Goldenrod Leaf
½ cup Gravel Root
½ cup Hydrangea Root
1 cup Uva Ursi Leaf
½ cup White Oak Bark
1 cup Parsley Leaf
½ cup Stinging Nettle Leaf
½ cup Tansy Flowers
1 cup Yellow Dock Root

"I only look for good in every life situation."

EXCEPTIONAL RELEASE
Support for the Bladder

1 cup Juniper Berries
1 cup Buchu Leaf
1 cup Celery Seeds
½ cup Fennel Seeds
1 cup Parsley Leaf
¼ cup Borage Leaf
1 cup Corn Silk
1 cup Uva Ursi Leaf
1 Quart Cranberry Juice
½ cup Dandelion Leaf
1 cup Goldenrod Leaf
½ cup Echinacea Leaf
½ cup Horsetail Leaf
¼ cup Lemon Balm Leaf

"Releasing toxic emotions is easy for me now."

EXPRESSION
Support for the Throat

1 cup Peppermint Leaf
½ Spearmint Leaf
½ cup Ginger Root
½ cup Slippery Elm Bark
½ cup Licorice Root
½ cup Marshmallow Root
½ cup Honeysuckle Flowers
1 cup Horehound Leaf
¼ cup Sage Leaf
LOTS OF RAW HONEY!

"I speak only my truth with love and sweetness."

*Additional Note:
Horehound Syrup can be used here for those who cannot tolerate certain sweeteners.

Ingredients:
½ cup horehound (flowering tops)
2 cups water
2 cups local raw honey (adjust to taste)

FEARLESSNESS
Support for Heartburn

½ cup Slippery Elm Bark
1 cup Fennel Seed
½ cup Anise Seed
1 cup Peppermint Leaf
1 cup Chamomile Flowers
1 cup Thyme Leaf
1 cup Marshmallow Leaf
½ cup Wood Betony Leaf

"I allow my heart to be at peace"

FERTILE GROUND
Support for Fertility

1 cup Red Raspberry Leaf
1 cup Dong Quai Root
½ cup False Unicorn Leaf
½ cup Damiana Leaf
¼ cup Oat Straw
1 cup Nettle Leaf
¼ cup Dandelion Leaf
¼ cup Alfalfa Leaf
¼ cup Red Clover Leaf
¼ cup Maca Root
¼ cup Vitex/Chaste Tree Berries
¼ cup Tribulus Berries

"I now lay fertile ground for new life."

FINE ALIGN
Support for Allergies

1 cup Chamomile Flowers
1 cup Echinacea Leaf
1 cup Stinging Nettles Leaf
1 cup Plantain Leaf
¼ cup Butterbur Leaf
½ cup Astralagus Leaf
¼ cup Ephedra Leaf
½ cup Thyme Leaf

"I claim my Divine power within me."

FLOW FREE

Support as an Anticoagulant

¼ cup Cayenne Pepper
1 cup Pennywort Leaf
½ cup Turmeric Root
1 cup Alfalfa Leaf
½ cup Angelica Leaf
¼ cup Anise Seed
¼ cup Arnica Leaf
½ cup Celery Seed
Juice bulb of Garlic

"My life force flows freely."

FLOW OF JOY
Support for High Cholesterol

1 cup Basil Leaf

1 cup Celery Seed

½ cup Fennel Seed

1 cup Parsley Leaf

½ cup Turmeric Root

1 cup Artichoke Leaf

1 cup Alfalfa Leaf

1 Whole Bulb Garlic

1 cup Echinacea Leaf

"I flow with the ever present joy of life."

FLU-AWAY
Support for Flu

1 cup Mullein Leaf
1 cup Sage Leaf
1 cup Elder Berry
1 cup Slippery Elm Bark
1 Whole Bulb Garlic
1 ½ Echinacea Leaf
1 cup Yarrow Leaf
½ cup Ginger Root
1 cup Buchu Leaf
½ cup Goldenseal Root
½ cup Licorice Root
½ cup Lemon Balm Leaf
½ cup Oregano Leaf
½ cup Thyme Leaf

"I claim my individual right to remain positive."

FREEDOM
Support for Addictions

1 cup Lemon Balm
2 cups Milk Thistle Seed
1 cup Agrimony
½ cup Licorice Root
½ cup Red Clover Leaf
½ cup Burdock Root
1 cup Dandelion Leaf
½ cup Yellow Dock Root
1 cup Peppermint Leaf
½ cup Kudzu Root
¼ cup Wormwood Leaf
½ cup Kava Kava Root
½ cup St John's Wort Leaf

"I am free, nothing has a hold over me."

FRESH FACE

Support for Acne

1 pint Aloe Juice (non-acidic)
1 cup Calendula Flowers
¼ Lavender Flowers
1 cup Walnut Leaf
1 cup Witch Hazel Leaf
½ cup Burdock Root
1 cup Milk Thistle Leaf
1 cup Buchu Leaf
¼ cup Chamomile Flowers
¼ cup Whole Cloves
¼ cupComfrey Root
½ cup Parsley Root

"I accept who I am in every way."

FULFILLED
Support for Yeast/Fungal Infections

½ cup Myrrh Gum
½ cup Black Walnut Bark
¼ cup Clove Bud
¼ cup Cinnamon
1 Quart Aloe Juice
1 cup Turmeric Root
1 cup Echinacea Leaf
½ cup Marigold Flowers
1 Whole Bulb Garlic
¼ cup Cayenne Pepper

"I release the past, it has no power over me now."

GERM-FREE

Support as an Antiseptic

1 cup Bergamot Leaf
1 cup Calendula Flowers
½ cup Cloves Bud
½ cup Ginger Root
¼ Lavender Flowers
1 cup Rose Hips Fruit
1 cup Yarrow Leaf

"I am at peace with love for who I am."

GOING VIRAL
Support as an Anti-Viral

Juice 2 bulbs Garlic
1 cup Oregano Leaf
1 cup Astralagus Leaf
1 cup Echinacea Root
1 cup Schizandra Berries
1 cup Elderberry
½ cup Licorice Root
½ cup Buchu Leaf
½ cup Goldenrod Leaf
½ cup Olive Leaf
¼ cup Juniper Berries
¼ cup Lemon Balm Leaf
¼ cup Shitake Mushroom
¼ cup Ginger Root
¼ cup Goldenseal Leaf
¼ cup St John's Wort
½ cup Echinacea Leaf
½ cup Rose Hips Fruit

"I trust the Universal supply."

GRACE AND EASE
Support for Joint Pain

1 cup Alfalfa Leaf
1 cup Black Cohosh Leaf
1 cup Bladderwrack Leaf
¼ cup Oregano Leaf
3 tbl Cayenne Pepper
1 cup Celery Seed
1 cup Red Clover Leaf
½ cup Comfrey Root
½ cup Devils Claw Leaf
¼ cup Ginger Root
¼ cup Lemon Grass
½ cup Parsley Leaf
¼ cup Stinging Nettles Leaf
¼ cup Turmeric Root
¼ cup Burdock Root
¼ cup Chaparral Leaf
¼ cup Wild Yam
½ cup White Willow Bark

"I move through life flexible and with ease."

GREAT CLEANSE
Support for Colon Cleanse

1 cup Blessed Thistle Leaf
1 cup Fenugreek Seed
1 cup Fennel Seed
½ cup Anise Seed
¼ cup Coriander Seed
¼ cup Spearmint Leaf
¼ cup Lemongrass Leaf
¼ cup Lemon Verbena Leaf
½ cup Marshmallow Leaf
1 cup Nettles Leaf
½ cup Alfalfa Leaf
¼ cup Caraway Seed

"I willingly release all stuck patterns."

HALO
Support for Scalp Issues

1 cup Rosemary Leaf
1 cup Stinging Nettles Leaf
½ cup Burdock Root
¼ cup Turmeric Root
½ cup Ginger Root
1 cup Sarsaparilla Root
½ cup Figwort Leaf
½ cup Oregon Grape Root
½ cup Yellow Dock Leaf
¼ cup Valerian Root
½ cup Skullcap Leaf

"I am crowned with glory and honor."

HAPPY BABY
Support for Colic

1 cup Bay Leaves
½ cup Anise Seed
½ cup Caraway Seed
½ cup Cardamom Seed
1 cup Catmint Leaf
1 cup Chamomile Flowers
½ cup Fennel Seed
½ cup Lemon Grass Leaf
½ cup Lemon Verbena Leaf
1 cup Lemon Balm Leaf
1 cup Peppermint Leaf
1 cup Rose Hips Fruit
1 cup Strawberry Leaf

"I am completely safe. I love being here."

*This mixture should be diluted ten parts or more of pure water to one part herbal mixture for babies. Discretion is necessary here.

HAPPY BELLY
Support for Pregnancy

1 cup Spearmint Leaf
1 cup Raspberry Leaf
¾ cup Strawberry Leaf
1 cup Nettle Leaf
½ cup Rose Hips Fruit
¼ cup Fennel Seed
¼ cup Lemongrass Leaf
1 cup Alfalfa Leaf
½ cup Lemon Verbena Leaf

"I bring forth new life with grace and ease."

HARMONY
Support for Incontinence

1 cup Buchu Leaf
1 cup Saw Palmetto Berries
¼ cup Cardamom Seeds
1 cup Corn Silk
½ cup Dandelion Leaf
½ cup Horsetail Leaf
1 cup Lemon Balm Leaf
1 cup Spearmint Leaf
½ cup Juniper Berries
½ cup Uva Ursi Leaf

"I now decide to let go of controlling my emptions. I am in the flow."

HAY-POWER
Support for Hay Fever

1 cup Butterbur Leaf
1 cup Stinging Nettles Leaf
½ cup Ginkgo Leaf
¼ cup Cinnamon Bark
1 cup Elderflowers
¼ cup Ephedra Powder
½ cup Eyebright Leaf
½ cup Ginkgo Leaf
1 cup Peppermint Leaf
½ cup Reishi Mushrooms
¼ cup Rosemary Leaf
1 cup Violet Leaf

"I am safe within the flow of my life."

HYDRATE ME
Support for Edema

1 cup Celery Seed
1 cup Raspberry Leaf
2 cups Corn Silk
1 cup Parsley Leaf
½ cup Fennel Seed
1 cup Alfalfa Leaf
1 cup Juniper Berries
½ cup Uva Ursi Leaf
1 cup Dandelion Leaf

"For my highest healing, I let of_____."

I LIVE
Support for Motion Sickness

1 cup Holy Basil Leaf
½ cup Fennel Seed
1 cup Peppermint Leaf
½ cup Thyme Leaf
½ cup Anise Seed
½ cup Fennel Seed
½ cup Ginger Root
1 cup Chamomile Flowers

"I am free."

I RELEASE
Support for Cramps

1 cup Cramp Bark
1 cup Peppermint Leaf
1 cup Alfalfa Leaf
½ cup Valerian Root
1 cup Skullcap Leaf
½ cup Yarrow Leaf
1 cup Chamomile Flowers
½ cup Calamus Leaf
½ cup Lavender Flowers
¼ cup Cinnamon Bark
¼ cup Red Peony Root
½ cup Chinese Motherwort Leaf
½ cup Chinese Angelica Leaf
¼ cup Szechuan Lovage Root

"I release into the process of life. Life happens well for me."

IN THE NIGHT
Support for Night Sweats

½ cup Dong Quai Root
¾ cup Black Cohosh Leaf
¼ cup Ginseng Root
½ cup Wild Yam Root
½ cup Red Clover Buds
½ cup Motherwort Leaf
½ cup Hops Flowers
¼ cup Sage Leaf
½ cup Vitex (Chaste Berries)
¼ cup Licorice Root
1 cup Alfalfa Leaf

"As anger rises to the surface, I gently release."

INSPIRE LIFE

Support for Bronchitis

½ cup Anise Seed
½ cup Cardamom Seed
1 cup Red Clover Leaf
1 cup Comfrey Leaf
1 cup Echinacea Leaf
1 cup Elderflower Leaf
½ cup Thyme Leaf
½ cup Mullein Leaf
¼ cup Anise Seed
½ cup Licorice Root
½ cup Nettle Leaf
¼ cup Caraway Seed
½ cup Coltsfoot Leaf
¼ cup Elecampane Leaf
½ cup Eucalyptus Leaf
½ cup Fennel Seed
½ cup Gingko Leaf
½ cup Honeysuckle Leaf

"My family environment is healing peacefully through me."

JOY IN THE MORNING
Support as an Anti-Depressant

¼ cup Damiana Leaf

½ cup Ginseng Leaf

½ cup Lady's Slipper Leaf

½ cup Saffron Leaf

½ cup Ginkgo Leaf

¼ cup Jasmine Flowers

¼ cup Lavender Flowers

¼ cup Lemon Verbena leaf

1 cup Oat Straw Leaf

½ cup Rosemary Leaf

¼ cup St John's Wort Leaf

"I am worthy of a beautiful life, I accept it now."

LISTEN NOW
Support for Coughs

1 cup Wild Cherry Bark
1 Pint Raw Honey
20 Squeezed Lemons
1 cup Slippery Elm Bark
1 cup Peppermint Leaf
1 cup Elderflower Leaf
½ cup Ginger Root
½ cup Elecampane Root
½ cup Slippery Elm Bark
½ cup Eucalyptus Leaf
1 cup Horehound Leaf
¼ cup Hyssop Leaf
¼ cup Pleurisy Root
1 cup Lemon Thyme Leaf
1 cup Mullein Flowers

"I speak distinctly, my wishes and I am clearly heard."

LOVIN LIFE!
Support for Gout

2 quarts Cherry Juice
2 cups Parsley Leaf
1 cup Stinging Nettle Leaf
1 cup Red Clover Leaf
½ cup Fennel Seed
½ cup Devils Claw Root
1 cup Celery Seed
1 cup Artichoke Leaf
½ cup Gravel Root (Kidneywort)
½ cup Turmeric Root
1 cup Alfalfa Leaf

"I submit to patience and joy."

NO CHILLS
Support for Chills

1 cup Echinacea Leaf
1 cup Ginger Root
1 cup Alfalfa Leaf
12 Squeezed Lemons

"I desire to stay in the present moment."

NO PRESSURE
Support for High Blood Pressure

1 cup Gingko Leaf
1 cup Hawthorn Berries
¼ cup Siberian Ginseng Root
Juice bulb Garlic
1 cup Maitake Mushroom
1 cup Olive Leaf
½ cup Basil Leaf
½ cup Celery Seeds
1 cup Yarrow Leaf

"I now choose to resolve deep-seated emotional issues."

PAID UP!
Support for Pain

1 cup Chamomile Leaf
¼ cup Clove Bud
1 cup Oat Straw
1 cup St John's Wort
½ cup Valerian Root
¼ cup Skullcap Leaf
½ cup Hops Flowers
1 cup Peppermint Leaf
1 cup Spearmint Leaf
½ cup Lemon Grass
½ cup Comfrey Root
¼ cup Kava Kava Root
¼ cup Ginger Root
¼ cup Eucalyptus Leaf
½ cup Turmeric Powder
1 cup White Willow Bark
1 cup Hops Flowers
½ cup Boswelia Resin (Frankincense)
½ cup Cat's Claw Root

"Everything I thought I owed, is now ALL paid up I owe nothing."

PH7
Support for Acidity

1 cup Chamomile Flowers
1 cup Fennel Seed
1 cup Marshmallow Root
1 cup Spearmint Leaf
2 cups Peppermint Leaf
½ cup Anise Seed
¼ cup Bay Leaves

"I am balanced with life."

POTENT

Support for Impotence

1 cup Ginkgo Leaf
1 cup Yohimbe Bark
1 cup Panax Ginseng Root
1 cup Muira Puama Root
1 cup Damiana Leaf
½ cup Fo-ti Root
½ cup Tongkat Ali Root
¼ cup Maca Root
½ cup Horny Goat Weed
¼ cup Tribulus Leaf
½ cup False Unicorn Leaf
½ cup Guarana Leaf
¼ cup Ashwagandha Root
½ cup Saw Palmetto Berries
¼ cup Pygeum Bark

"I express generously through my sexual energy."

PROCESS
Support for Rashes

1 cup Calendula Flowers
½ cup Comfrey Root
1 cup Elder Flower
½ cup Red Clover Leaf
1 Quart Aloe Juice (non-acidic)
½ cup Milk Thistle Seeds
1 cup Dandelion Leaf
½ cup Burdock Root
1 cup Alfalfa Leaf
1 cup Yellow Dock Leaf

"I am patient with the processes of life."

PROSPEROUS
Support for Fungal Infections

½ cup Myrrh Gum
½ cup Black Walnut Bark
¼ cup Clove Bud
¼ cup Cinnamon Bark
1 Quart Aloe Juice
1 cup Turmeric Root
1 cup Echinacea Leaf
½ cup Marigold Flowers
1 Whole Bulb Garlic
3 tbl Cayenne Pepper

"I release and let the present moment rule."

PURE JOY
Support for Arthritis

1 cup Alfalfa Leaf
1 cup Black Cohosh Leaf
1 cup Bladderwrack Leaf
¼ cup Oregano Leaf
3 tbls Cayenne Pepper
1 cup Celery Leaf
1 cup Red Clover Leaf
½ cup Comfrey Root
½ cup Devils Claw Leaf
¼ cup Ginger Root
¼ cup Lemon Grass
½ cup Parsley Leaf
¼ cup Stinging Nettles Leaf
¼ cup Turmeric Root
¼ cup Burdock Root
¼ cup Chaparral Leaf
¼ cup Wild Yam Root
½ cup White Willow Bark

"My joy has moved my heart to sing.

PURITY
Support as an Antibiotic

Juice bulb of Garlic
Juice 12 Lemons
1 cup Goldenseal Leaf
½ cup Bladderwrack Leaf
1 cup Buchu Leaf
1 cup Echinacea Leaf
½ cup Echinacea Root
1 cup Alfalfa Leaf
¼ cup Rosemary Leaf
¼ cup Sage

"I purify my mind and my heart with love."

QUALITY FLOW I
Support for Increased Breast Milk

1 cup Blessed Thistle Leaf
1 cup Fenugreek Seed
1 cup Fennel Seed
½ cup Anise Seed
¼ cup Coriander Seed
¼ cup Spearmint Leaf
¼ cup Lemongrass Leaf
¼ cup Lemon Verbena Leaf
½ cup Marshmallow Leaf
1 cup Nettles Leaf
½ cup Alfalfa Leaf
¼ cup Caraway Seeds

"I increase my flow of love to my newborn."

QUALITY FLOW II
Support for Decreased Breast Milk

1 cup Peppermint Leaf
1 cup Spearmint Leaf
1 cup Parsley Leaf
1 cup Chickweed Leaf
½ cup Black Walnut Leaf
1 cup Yarrow Leaf
¼ cup Lemon Balm Leaf

"I flow my love to other areas of my child's life."

RECESS
Support as an Anti-Spasmodic

¼ cup Anise Seed
½ cup Basil Leaf
¼ cup Cardamom Seed
1 cup Chamomile Flowers
¼ Cinnamon Bark
¼ cup Cloves Bud
½ cup Lemon Thyme Leaf
½ cup Lemon Verbena Leaf
½ cup Marjoram Leaf
½ Lemon Balm Leaf
¼ cup Rosemary Leaf
½ cup St John's Wort Leaf
1 cup Yarrow Leaf

"I relax and let flow happen."

RECOGNITION
Support for Nosebleed

1 cup Bilberry Leaf
1 cup Nettle Leaf
¼ cup Cayenne Pepper
1 cup Raspberry Leaf
1 cup Witch Hazel Leaf
¼ cup Comfrey Root
½ cup Parsley Leaf
¼ cup Agrimony Leaf
¼ cup Yarrow Leaf

"I recognize and embrace the love I feel for me."

REGENERATION
Support for Thyroid

1 cup Echinacea Leaf
¼ cup Licorice Root
¼ cup Bugleweed Leaf
½ cup Siberian Ginseng Root
½ cup Bladderwrack Leaf
¼ cup Black Walnut Leaf
½ cup Lemon Balm
¼ Ashwagandha Root
½ cup Schizandra Berries

"I am regenerating now."

REJUVENATION
Support for Exhaustion

2 cups Alfalfa Leaf
1 cup Oat Straw
½ cup Peppermint Leaf
½ cup Rosemary Leaf
1 cup Gotu Kola Leaf
1 cup Guarana Leaf
2 tbls Cayenne Pepper
1 cup Ginkgo Leaf
1 cup Siberian Ginseng Leaf
½ cup Ashwaganda Leaf
½ cup Astragalus Leaf
½ cup Stinging Nettle Leaf
¼ cup Reishi Mushroom

"I am rejuvenating now."

RESPONSIBILITY
Support for Psoriasis

2 Quarts Aloe Juice (non-acidic)
1 cup Calendula Flowers
½ cup Evening Primrose Root or Flowers
1 cup Neem Leaf
1 cup Milk Thistle Seeds
½ cup Dandelion Leaf
½ cup Burdock Root
½ cup Oregon Grape Root
½ cup Red Clover Leaf
½ cup Turmeric Root
1 cup Parsley Leaf

"I enliven all my sense and take FULL responsibility for my feelings right now."

RESTORATION
Support for Hormonal Balance

1 cup Red Clover Leaf
1 cup Black Cohosh Leaf
1 cup Dong Quai Root
½ Licorice Root
1 cup Damiana Leaf
1 cup Vitex Leaf
¼ Hops Flowers
¼ Ginseng Root
½ cup Ginkgo Leaf
½ cup Chaste Tree Leaf
1 cup False Unicorn Root
½ cup Sage Leaf
1 cup Raspberry Leaf
½ St John's Wort Leaf
1 cup Sarsaparilla Leaf
½ cup Saw Palmetto Berries
½ cup Shepard's Purse Leaf
½ cup True Unicorn Bark
¼ cup Wild Yam Bark

"I am restoring the proper balance to my life."

RIGHT TIME
Support for Hemorrhoids

¼ cup Horse Chestnut Leaf
1 cup Bilberry Leaf
1 cup Chamomile Flowers
1 cup Plantain Leaf
1 cup Butchers Broom Leaf
Quart of Aloe Juice (non-acidic)
1 cup Horsetail Leaf
1 cup Dandelion Leaf
½ cup St John's Wort Leaf
1 cup Peppermint Leaf
1 cup Spearmint Leaf

"I am right on time to let go of the burdens of fear from the past."

SATIETY
Support for Lack of Appetite

1 cup Ginger Root
2 cup Blessed Thistle Leaf
2 cups Peppermint Leaf
1 tbl Nutmeg
1 tsp Cinnamon
1 Quart Fresh Pressed Apple Juice
12 Lemons

"I bless the healing power of food."

SELFLESS
Support for Nerves

1 cup Mullein Leaf
1 cup Sage Leaf
1 cup Elderberry
1 cup Slippery Elm Bark
1 Whole Bulb Garlic
1 ½ Echinacea Leaf
1 cup Yarrow Leaf
½ cup Ginger Root
1 cup Buchu Leaf
½ cup Goldenseal Root
½ cup Licorice Root
½ cup Lemon Balm Leaf
½ cup Oregano Leaf
½ cup Thyme Leaf

"I indulge in communication about how I feel."

SHEER DELIGHT
Support for Urinary Tract Infection

1 cup Celery Seed
½ cup Fennel Seed
2 cups Corn Silk
2 cups Parsley Leaf
1 cup Spearmint Leaf
1 Quart Pure Cranberry Juice
½ cup Horseradish grated
1 cup Marshmallow Leaf
¼ cup Uva Ursi Leaf
¼ cup St. John's Wort Leaf
¼ cup Horsetail Leaf
¼ cup Dandelion Root
¼ cup Yellow Root
1 cup Echinacea Leaf
½ cup Nettles Leaf

"Life is a sheer delight and I am happy with my life partners."

SINUS SOOTHING
Support for Sinus Issues

1 cup Eucalyptus Leaf
¼ cup Licorice Root
¼ cup Horseradish Root grated
½ cup Nettle Leaf
1 cup Peppermint Leaf
½ cup Ginger Root grated
½ cup Echinacea Root
¼ cup Golden Seal Root
1 cup Elder Berry
½ cup Fenugreek Seed
½ cup Thyme Leaf
¼ cup Juniper Berries
½ cup Calendula Flowers
¼ cup Myrrh Bark
1 tablespoon Cayenne Pepper (or to taste)

"I am agreeable with all those around me."

SOFT SKIN
Support for Dry Skin

1 cup Borage Leaf
1 cup Dandelion Leaf
1 cup Milk Thistle Seed
1 cup Calendula Flowers
½ cup Lady's Mantle Flowers
1 cup Marshmallow Leaf
1 cup Lemon Balm Leaf
½ cup Clary Sage Leaf

"I feel comfortable in my skin."

SOOTHE AND EASE
Support as an Analgesic

1 cup Chamomile Flowers
½ Goldenseal Leaf
1 cup Licorice Root
1 cup Marshmallow Leaf
1 cup Slippery Elm Bark

"I ease my body into peace and calm."

SOPHISTICATED LADY
Support for PMS

1 cup False Unicorn Root
1 cup Damiana Leaf
2 cups Red Raspberry Leaf
½ cup Fo-Ti Root
½ cup Wild Yam Root
½ cup Chasteberry (Vitex)
¼ cup Black Cohosh Leaf
½ cup Dong Quai Root
¼ cup St. John's Wort
¼ cup Maca Root
¼ cup Burdock Root
¼ cup Lemon Balm Leaf
¼ cup Ginkgo Leaf
¼ cup Thyme Leaf
¼ cup Ginger Root
¼ cup Cinnamon Bark

"I am clear, powerful and satisfied with my feminine nature."

SOVEREIGNTY
Support for Parasites

1 cup Black Walnut
½ cup Cloves
1 cup Ginger Root
3 tbls Cayenne
¼ cup Golden Seal Root
½ cup Oregon Grape Root
1 cup Wormwood
½ cup Thyme Leaf
½ cup Barberry
½ cup Gentian Root
½ cup Oregano Leaf
Juice of Whole Bulb Garlic
Juice of Large Red Onion

"I have full power over my life."

STERILE AND FREE
Support as an Anti-Bacterial

½ cup Oregon Grape Root
½ cup Turmeric Root
1 cup Calendula Flowers
¼ cup Cinnamon Bark
½ cup Lavender Flowers
¼ cup Marjoram Leaf
1 cup Witch Hazel Leaf

"Only purity lives within me."

STIMULATE
Support as a Stimulator

1 cup Rosemary Leaf
¼ cup Clove Bud
½ cup Ginger Root
½ cup Siberian Ginseng Root
¼ cup Cayenne Pepper
¼ cup Nutmeg
½ cup Angelica Root
1 cup Guarana Leaf
1 cup Ginkgo Leaf

"I am stimulated to achieve great things!"

SWEET BALANCE
Support as a Diuretic

1 cup Celery Seed

1 cup Corn Silk

1 cup Parsley Leaf

1 cup Stinging Nettle Leaf

½ cup Sage Leaf

¼ cup Hops Flower

¼ cup Fennel Seed

¼ cup Chicory Mint Leaf

½ cup Yarrow Leaf

¼ cup Goldenseal Root

½ cup Dandelion Leaf

1 cup Nettle Leaf

½ cup Marshmallow Leaf

1 cup Spearmint Leaf

½ cup Linden Flower

1 cup Artichoke Leaf

1 cup Goldenrod Leaf

¼ cup Chamomile Flowers

½ cup Corn Silk

"I feel lifted, light and balanced."

SWEET FEET
Support for Athlete's Foot

1 cup Buchu Leaf
1 cup Calendula Flowers
½ cup Olive Leaf
1 cup Pau D Arco Leaf
½ cup Goldenseal Root
1 cup Witch Hazel Leaf
1 cup White Oak Bark
¼ cup Thyme Leaf
1 cup Goldenseal Leaf
1 cup Echinacea Root
1 cup Echinacea Leaf

"The path is clear for my new walk."

SWEET INDULGENCE
Support for Anorexia

¼ cup Cardamom Seed
Juice 1 bulb Garlic
½ cup Ginger Root
½ cup Thyme Leaf
2 cups Alfalfa Leaf
1 cup Yarrow Leaf
1 cup Peppermint Leaf
½ cup Fennel Seed
½ cup Hyssop Leaf
½ cup Dandelion Leaf
½ cup Wormwood Leaf
½ cup Fenugreek Seed
½ cup Lemon Balm Leaf
½ cup Chamomile Flowers

"I allow myself to enjoy all of life's delights today!"

THE RIGHT CHARGE
Support for Prostate

1 cup Corn Silk
½ cup Bitter Melon Seeds
1 cup Raspberry Leaf
1 cup Plantain Leaf
1 cup Saw Palmetto Berries
½ cup Red Clover Leaf
½ cup Pygueum Bark
1 cup Stinging Nettles Leaf
1 cup Uva Ursi Leaf

"I am Just Right."

TIMELESSNESS
Support for Anti-Aging

1 cup Gingko Leaf
1 cup Gotu Kola Leaf
1 cup Artichoke Leaf
½ cup Milk Thistle Leaf
½ cup Dandelion Leaf
½ cup Saw Palmetto Fruit
½ cup Black Cohosh Leaf
½ cup Juniper Berries
½ cup Buchu Leaf
½ cup Hawthorn Berries
½ cup Burdock Root
1 cup Peppermint Leaf
¼ cup Chamomile Flowers
Pinch of Cayenne Pepper
Juice bulb of Garlic
½ cup Celery Leaf
¼ cup Lemon Thyme Leaf
1 cup Alfalfa Leaf

"Timelessness is a blessing."

TOLERANCE
Support for Jaundice

1 cup Dandelion Leaf
½ cup Silverweed
1 Quart Black Radish Juice
½ cup Milk Thistle Seed
1 cup Artichoke Leaf
1 cup St John's Wort Leaf
½ cup Blackthorn Tree
¼ cup Fennel Seeds
½ cup Stinging Nettles Leaf
¼ cup Horsetail Leaf
¼ cup Chamomile Flowers
¼ cup Angelica Root

"Everything I see is in Divine Order, I can simply choose to like it."

ULTIMATE CLEANSE
Support for Liver

1 cup Dandelion Leaf
1 cup Milk Thistle Seeds
½ cup Oregon Grape Root
1 cup Burdock Root
1 cup Red Clover Leaf
1 cup Yellow Dock Leaf
½ cup Licorice Root
1 cup Celery Seed
1 cup Echinacea Leaf
1 cup Hyssop Leaf
½ cup Goldenseal Root
¼ cup Cayenne Pepper
1 cup Peppermint Leaf
½ cup Cascara Sagrada Bark
½ cup Fennel Seed
1 Quart Aloe Juice (non-acidic)
½ cup Thyme Leaf
½ cup Fenugreek Seed
12 Squeezed Lemons

"I transform my anger into joy."

VALUABLE CURRENCY
Support for Circulation

1 cup Ginger Root
1 cup Ginkgo Leaf
¼ cup Cayenne Pepper
1 cup Rosemary Leaf
½ cup Gotu Kola Leaf
½ cup Rosemary Leaf
1 cup Yarrow Leaf
1 cup Hawthorn Berries
1 Whole Bulb Garlic
¼ cup Horse Chestnut Leaf

"I flow with the currency of gratitude."

VERY FITTING
Support for Weight Loss

1 cup Sarsaparilla Bark
¼ cup Licorice Root
1 cup Corn Silk
¼ cup Horehound Leaf
½ cup Kelp
½ cup Bladderwrack
½ cup Echinacea Leaf
1 cup Chickweed Leaf
¼ cup Burdock Root
¼ cup Black Walnut Hulls
1 cup Cleavers Leaf
½ cup Yerba Mate Leaf
½ cup Plantain Leaf
1 cup Spearmint Leaf
½ cup Oat Straw

"I allow others to align with the goodness that I am."
*Optional: You can add a quart of pure Cranberry Juice
or/and a quart of Fresh Pressed Aloe Juice (non-acidic)

VISIONS
Support for the Eyes

½ cup Fennel Seeds
1 cup Eyebright Leaf
½ cup Ginkgo Root
¼ cup Milk Thistle Seeds
¼ cup Saffron Powder
1 cup Bilberry Leaf
½ cup Anise Seed
1 cup Passionflower

"I can see clearly now."

*Additional info for eyes: Bentonite Clay, Chickweed and Fennel poultice will work wonders in both removing toxins and soothing the eyes. Eyebright still works wonders as a eyewash.

VITAL CLEANSE
Support for Blood

1 cup Burdock Root
1 cup Basil Leaf
1 cup Echinacea Root
1 cup Echinacea Leaf
1 cup Red Clover Leaf
1 cup Alfalfa Leaf
½ cup Dandelion Root
½ cup Yellowdock Leaf

"My flow of life is pure."

WELLBEING*FEMALE
Support for Female

1 cup False Unicorn Root
1 cup Damiana Leaf
2 cups Red Raspberry Leaf
½ cup Fo-Ti Root
½ cup Wild Yam Root
1 cup Catnip Leaf
1 cup Echinacea Leaf
½ cup Hyssop Leaf
¼ cup Licorice Root
¼ cup Thyme Leaf
½ cup Elder Flower
¼ cup Ginger Root
¼ cup Lemon Grass
½ cup Yarrow Leaf
1 tbl Cayenne Pepper
¼ cup Cinnamon Bark
3 tbl Clove Bud

"I choose love, abundance, peace, clarity and wealth of health."

WELLBEING*MALE
Support for Male

1 cup Hawthorn Berries
1 cup Maca Root
1 cup Siberian Ginseng Root
½ cup American Ginseng Root
½ cup Ashwagandha Root
¼ cup Ginger Root
½ cup Ginkgo Root
½ cup Damiana Leaf
¼ cup Cinnamon Bark
¼ cup Horny Goat Weed
¼ cup Kava Kava Root
¼ cup Muira Puama Bark
½ cup Oat Straw
1 cup Sarsaparilla Bark
½ cup Saw Palmetto Berries
½ cup Yohimbe Bark
½ cup Astragalus Root
¼ cup Cordyceps Mushroom
¼ cup Reishi Mushroom
¼ cup Deer Antler

"I affirm only the best for my life"

WHOLE AGAIN
Support for Bone Fracture

1 cup Comfrey Root
1 Quart Aloe Juice
1 cup Peppermint Leaf
1 cup Horsetail Leaf
¼ cup Turmeric Root
½ cup Cactus Leaf
½ cup Marshmallow Leaf

"I allow wholeness."

WITH A CHILD'S HEART
Support for Low Blood Pressure

1 cup Rosemary Leaf
1 cup Motherwort Leaf
1 cup Hawthorn Berries
½ cup Ginger Root
1 cup Ginseng Root
1 cup Siberian Ginseng Root
½ cup Scotch Broom Leaf or Flower
½ cup Indian Spikeard Leaf
1 cup Nettle Leaf

"Nothing's gonna get me down."

WORKOUT
Support for Torn Ligaments

1 cup Horsetail Leaf
1 cup Devils Claw Root
1 cup Comfrey Root
2 Quarts Aloe Juice (non-acidic)
1 cup Peppermint Leaf
1 cup Pennywort Leaf

"I am bringing it all back together in my life."

ABOUT THE AUTHOR

Ombassa Sophera was initiated into the health and wellness field through her love and commitment to find options for ultimate health and well-being for her family. After years of study and providing health empowerment events, she began facilitating her signature workshop in 1997, **"Taking Responsibility for Your Health and Well-Being"**. Since then, she has combined years of experience and study with her innate gifts and abilities, assisting clients who seek solutions to the spiritual, emotional, mental and physical health issues that cause imbalances in their lives.

Ombassa is the author of Soul Journey to Truth, a book of poetry and affirmations, now in its 3rd edition.

www.ombassa.com